H1N1 FLU

A GUIDE FOR COMMUNITY
-AND-
FAITH-BASED ORGANIZATIONS

This document was produced by the
Center for Faith-based and Neighborhood Partnerships at the
U.S. Department of Health and Human Services with support from the Centers for Disease Control and Prevention

TABLE OF CONTENTS

Dear Friends,

Thank you for your leadership and the compassionate service you provide to your communities. People often turn to community and faith-based organizations to get the most up-to-date information on health and other important community issues. You have a unique ability to reach deeply into your community and connect people with the information and resources they need to help stay healthy.

My colleagues at HHS and I will continue to do everything in our power to help keep Americans healthy and safe this flu season. But government cannot respond alone. That is why I am pleased to present *"H1N1 Flu: A Guide for Community and Faith-Based Organizations."* Inside, you'll find information about how your community or faith-based organization can:

· Ensure information is communicated effectively, accurately, and with cultural sensitivity to community members,

· Help those who are most vulnerable and hard-to-reach,

· Partner with local governments to assist in vaccine distribution, and

· Adjust activities in ways that will help protect your community from flu.

This flu season, you will play a vital role in our country's national preparedness and response efforts. Thank you for your partnership as we work together this fall to help keep our communities healthy.

Sincerely

Kathleen Sebelius
Secretary
Department of Health and Human Services

To help keep communities healthy during the upcoming flu season, it will take all of us— community and faith-based organizations, government, businesses, and schools—working together. The federal government alone cannot prepare for or respond to the challenge of the 2009-2010 flu season.

Leaders and members of community and faith-based organizations (CFBOs), people like you, know their communities well. As trusted leaders, you can communicate important health information in an effective and motivating manner. You know the people in your community who are most vulnerable and hard-to-reach. Organizations like yours are uniquely positioned to help keep people healthy during the 2009-2010 flu season.

In addition to providing information about 2009 H1N1 flu and current response activities, this guide provides specific action steps you can take to help keep your community healthy by:

- **Communicating health information effectively;**

- **Supporting vaccination efforts;**

- **Linking vulnerable and hard-to-reach populations to vital information and resources; and**

- **Expanding and adjusting organizational activities to help people stay healthy.**

Since there is a great deal of variation among CFBOs, different parts of this document will be more relevant to your organization than others. Use this guide to help inform your response to both 2009-2010 seasonal and 2009 H1N1 flu. Remember to be creative as you design a response plan that is relevant and useful to the people you serve.

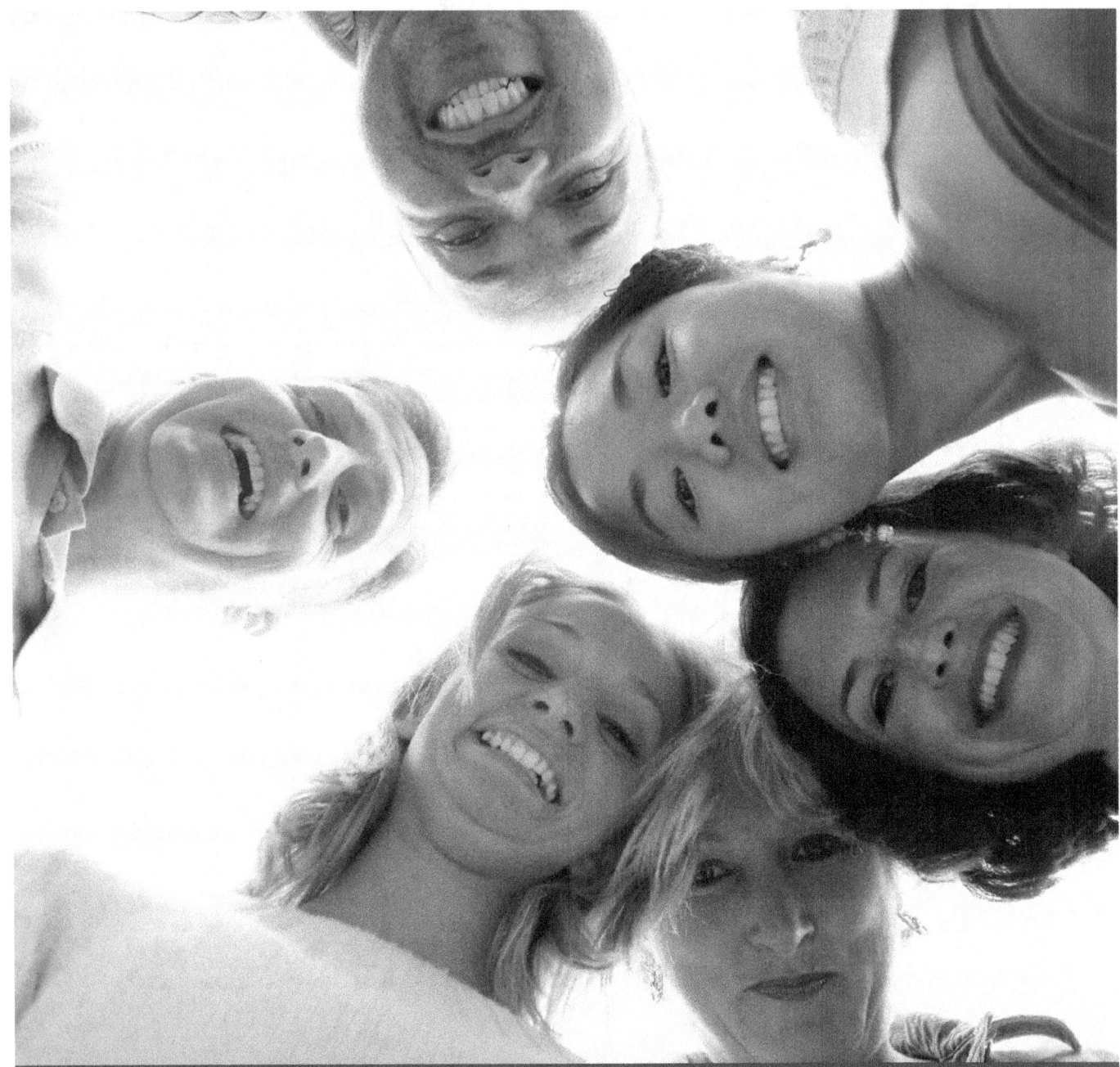

BOX 1: 2009 H1N1 Vaccine Target Groups

- Pregnant women
- Household contacts and caregivers for children younger than 6 months old
- Healthcare and emergency medical services personnel
- All people from 6 months through 24 years of age
- People aged 25 through 64 years with chronic health conditions (including asthma, heart disease, diabetes, HIV, and other disorders)

Community and Faith-based Involvement

What can CFBOs do to help people stay healthy during the 2009-2010 flu season?

- **Spread the word** about what individuals can do to prepare for and stay healthy during the 2009-2010 flu season. Check **http://www.flu.gov for the most up-to-date information on current recommendations.** (See Appendix A for more details.)

- **Work closely with your local or state health department to educate community members on flu.** For example, your organization could:
  - Institute a "Healthy Habits" or "Flu Facts" section in your newsletter;
  - Sponsor a community lecture series on preventing and treating flu; or
  - Develop a "buddy" system to help ensure vulnerable and hard-to-reach community members stay connected to flu-related news and services.

- **Support state and local health departments' vaccination efforts by:**
  - Encouraging community members to get vaccinated for seasonal flu;
  - Helping people to understand the initial target groups for 2009 H1N1 flu (see Box 1);
  - Encouraging these groups to get the 2009 H1N1 flu vaccination;
  - Providing facilities as vaccination sites in partnership with your state or local health department;
  - Providing information about where vaccine is available; and
  - Tailoring health department information on vaccinations to meet the specific cultural or religious needs of your community.

    Note: See Section B on vaccine distribution for more information.

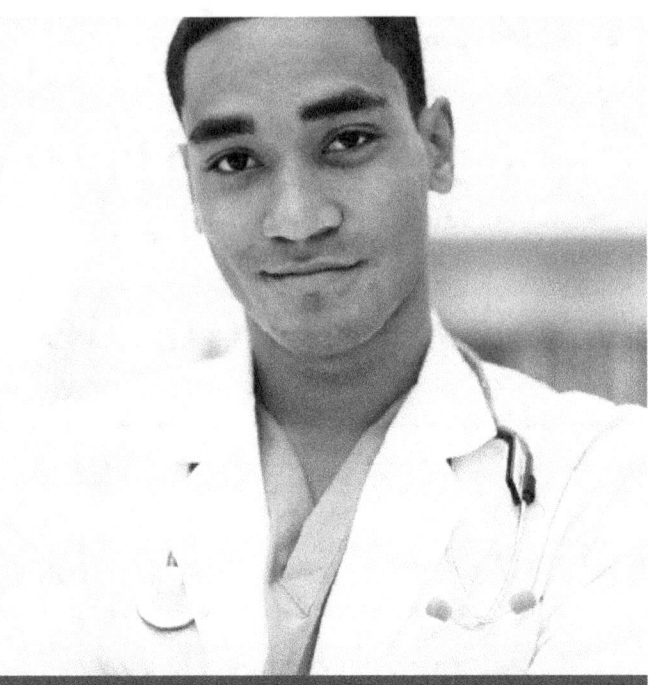

- Encourage individuals and families to be prepared for 2009 HlNl flu by:

  - Practicing Healthy Habits (see Box 2);

  - Staying up-to-date on immunizations, including getting the seasonal flu vaccine and the 2009 HlNl flu vaccine, if recommended;

  - Keeping a current list of medical conditions and medications;

  - Checking and refilling supplies of regular prescription and over-the-counter drugs periodically to ensure an adequate supply; and

  - Maintaining a two-week supply of food and other necessities to avoid the need to shop while you are sick or if local businesses are closed because illness is widespread in your community. See http://www.flu.gov/plan/individual/checklist.html for a checklist.

How can my organization create effective partnerships for the 2009-2010 flu season?

Your organization does not need to do everything on its own. Here are a few steps your organization can take to help ensure a coordinated response:

- **Work with your state, local, tribal, or territorial government** to coordinate with other national and local response efforts in your community.

- **Partner with organizations within your existing associations and networks.**

BOX 2: Practice Healthy Habits During Flu Season

- Cover your nose and mouth with a tissue when you cough or sneeze. Throw the tissue in the trash after you use it. If a tissue is unavailable, cough or sneeze into your shoulder or elbow instead of your hands.

- Wash your hands often or use hand sanitizer.

- Avoid touching your eyes, nose, or mouth.

- Get the seasonal flu vaccine and/or the 2009 HlNl flu vaccine, if recommended (see Section B for more information on vaccine recommendations).

- Try to avoid close contact with sick people.

- Keep sick children at home.

- If you have flu-like symptoms (fever with cough or sore throat), stay home for at least 24 hours after you are free of fever without the use of fever-reducing medications.

Vaccine Distribution

When will the 2009 HINI flu vaccine be available?

The 2009 HINI flu vaccine is expected to be available in October.

Do I need both the seasonal flu vaccine and the 2009 HINI flu vaccine?

Yes, especially if you are in one of the target groups for the 2009 HINI flu vaccine.

Who should get the seasonal flu vaccine?

The seasonal flu vaccine is recommended for anyone who wants to reduce their risk of becoming ill with flu. It is particularly important for persons at increased risk of severe illness or for spreading the infection to persons who are at high risk. These people include:

- **People aged 6 months through 18 years or age 50 years or older;**

- **People with underlying medical conditions, such as chronic heart or lung diseases or diabetes (see Appendix A for a full list of these conditions);**

- **Pregnant women;**

- **Healthcare providers;**

- **People who live with or care for infants younger than 6 months of age; and**

- **Residents of long-term care facilities.**

If you are unsure about whether you should receive the seasonal flu vaccine, contact your healthcare provider.

What are the target groups for the 2009 HINI flu vaccine?

When the vaccine first becomes available, the groups of people who will be in greatest need for protection by vaccination with the 2009 HINI flu vaccine are:

- Pregnant women;

- Household contacts and caregivers for children younger than 6 months old;

- Healthcare and emergency medical services (EMS) personnel;

- All people aged 6 months to 24 years; and

- People aged 25 through 64 years with chronic health conditions (see Appendix A for a list of these medical conditions).

Healthcare and EMS personnel have been targeted for vaccination to keep them healthy, able to work, and less likely to infect their patients on the job. Other persons have been targeted for vaccination to protect them from medical complications if they get 2009 HINI flu.

Once the demand for vaccine in target groups has been met at the local level, programs and providers should also begin vaccinating everyone from the ages of 25 through 64 years.

Should senior citizens be vaccinated for 2009 HINI flu?

Based on what we know about 2009 HINI flu, people age 65 or older have a lower risk of being infected with 2009 HINI flu than younger people. However, the small minority of people over 65 who do become infected with HINI are at higher risk of complications. Therefore, any person over 65 who becomes ill with flu-like symptoms should contact his or her physician right away to determine whether treatment with antivirals is needed. Also, seniors should consider getting the 2009 HINI flu vaccine once the target groups mentioned above have been offered vaccine.

Where will the 2009 HINI flu vaccine be available?

Vaccine will likely be available in healthcare provider offices, health departments, schools, and other settings, including pharmacies, workplaces, and community centers. Every state is developing a vaccine delivery plan. For more information about obtaining the flu vaccine, contact your doctor or local health department. To find a clinic near you, visit http://www.flu.gov/individualfamily/vaccination/locator.html.

BOX 3: Promising Partnership— MINI Project

The Minnesota Immunization Networking Initiative (MINI) Project works to increase annual seasonal flu immunizations in the Twin Cities area, specifically among minority, immigrant, and uninsured populations. A collaborative effort between non-profit and for-profit organizations and corporations, government agencies, and faith communities, the MINI project has provided a total of 16,000 free immunizations at 52 multi-cultural clinic sites since the program's inception in 2006. The immunizations are administered by healthcare workers at non-traditional clinic sites, such as churches, mosques, and community centers, at times when people are present for other activities. See Appendix C if you are interested in setting up a similar partnership.

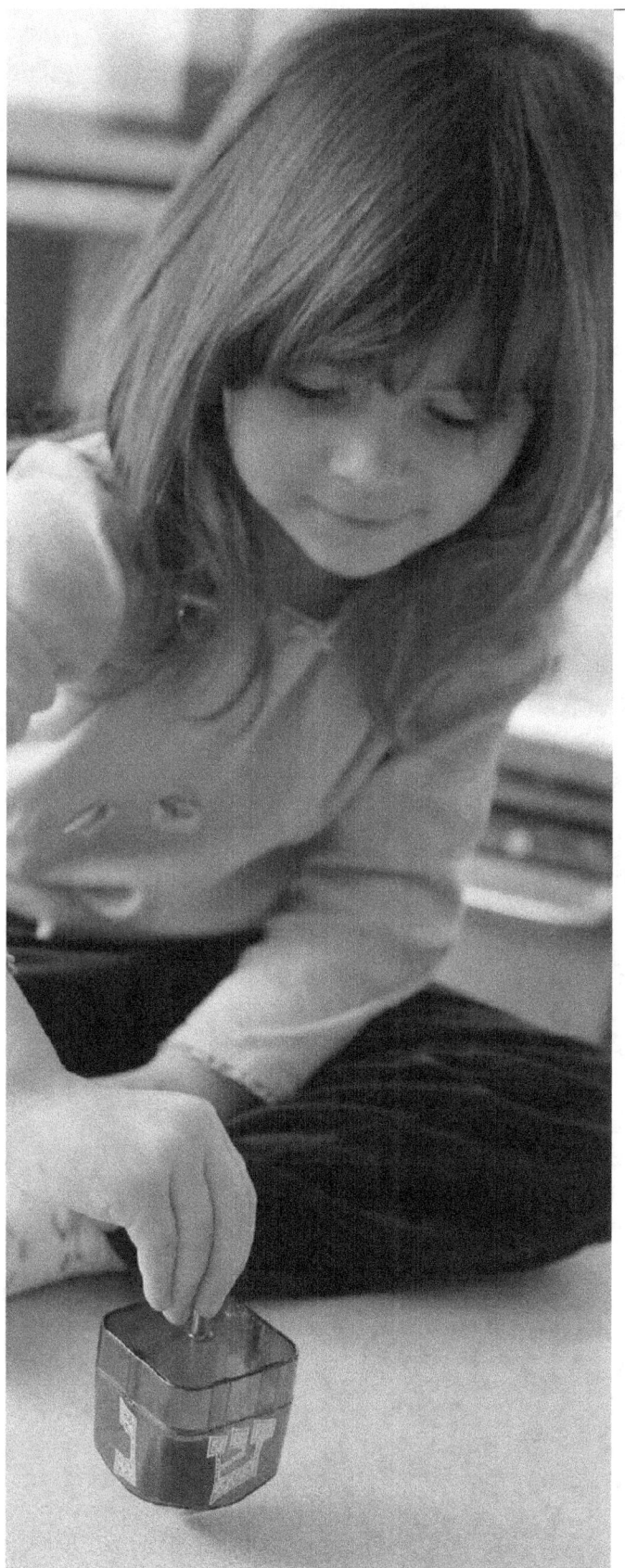

What about the use of antivirals to treat flu?

Antiviral drugs are prescription medicines (pills, liquid, or an inhaled powder) that help your body fight flu (both seasonal and 2009 H1N1). If you get sick with flu, antiviral drugs may make your illness milder and make you feel better faster. **If people at risk of medical complications from flu develop flu-like symptoms, they should seek treatment from a healthcare provider within 48 hours, including antiviral treatment.** For updated information on using antivirals during the 2009-2010 flu season, visit: http://www.cdc.gov/h1n1flu/antiviral.htm.

How can my organization support 2009 H1N1 flu vaccine distribution efforts?

- **Encourage community members to get vaccinated for seasonal and 2009 H1N1 flu** according to Centers for Disease Control and Prevention (CDC) recommendations. Here are a few ideas:
  - Include reminders to get vaccinated in regular communications and gatherings.
  - Hold an information session on flu vaccination for people in your community. Ask a health professional in your community or organization to give a presentation.
  - Provide community members with information on where and when they can go to get flu vaccinations. Check with your local health department to get this information.
  - Organize rides to vaccination clinics and/or set up vaccination appointments.
  - Help people understand vaccination target groups.

- **Follow up with community members** to help ensure that they receive all necessary vaccinations and see their doctor for treatment.

- **Offer your building or facilities as vaccination sites.** Work with your local health department to organize this effort. See Box 3 as an example of such a partnership.

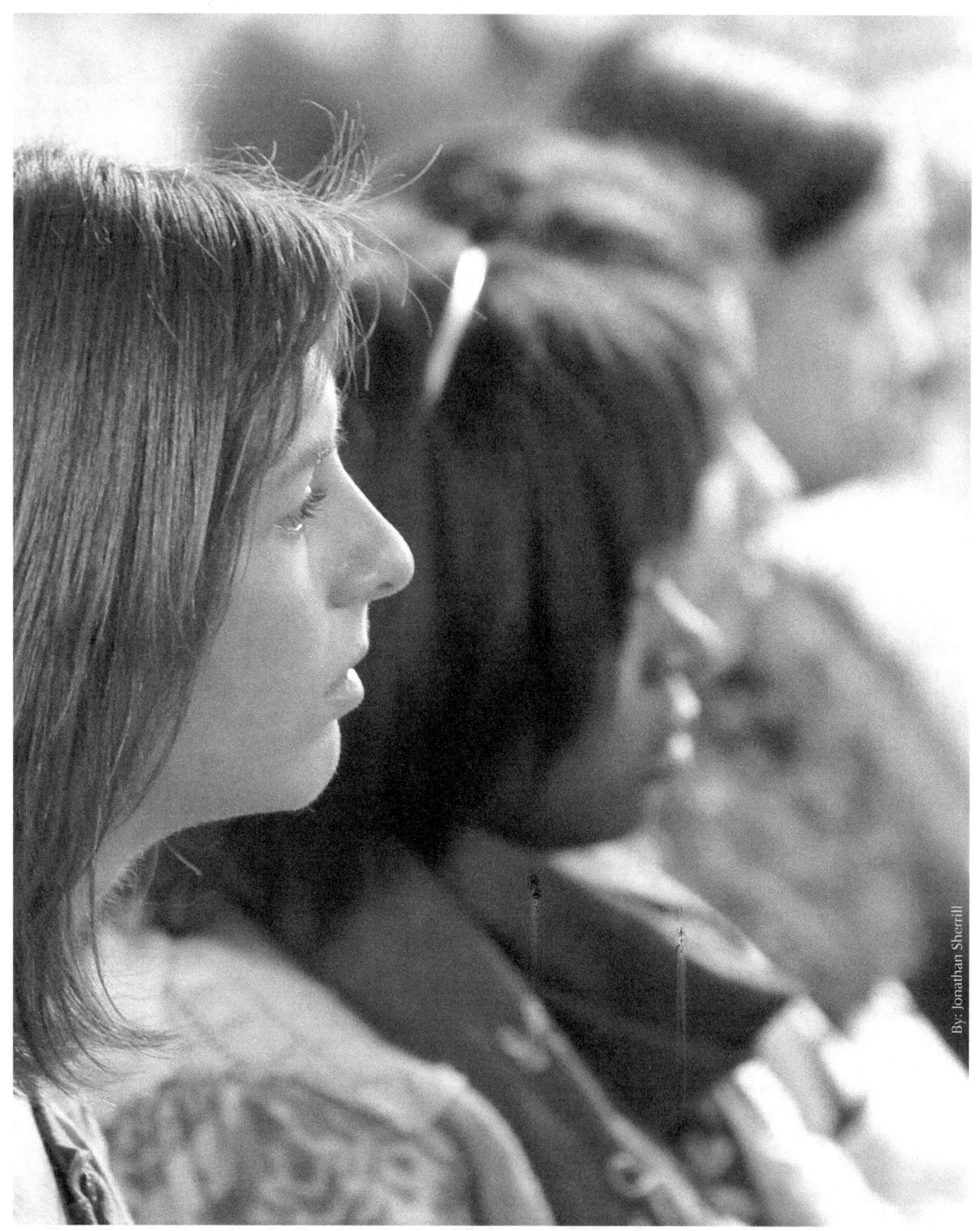

By: Jonathan Sherrill

Communication

How can my organization communicate effectively about flu?

Your organization can play a vital role in ensuring that accurate public health information is communicated effectively. When information is shared by trusted messengers, people are more likely to respond and change their behavior. We also need your help to deliver these public health messages to hard-to-reach people.

Here are some strategies for sharing messages:

- **Check http://www.flu.gov for the most up-to-date information,** and share what you learn with your faith community or organization.

- **Provide timely and accurate information.** You are uniquely positioned to share information with community members in both culturally appropriate and easy-to-understand ways.

- **Communicate and create linkages to populations that are vulnerable or hard-to-reach,** including people who are homeless, shut-in, low-income, non-English-speaking, unconnected to mainstream media, or are migrant workers, immigrants, or refugees. See Section D on vulnerable and hard-to-reach populations for more information.

- **Make sure that people can access your organization in alternate ways.** You might consider:
  - Organizing a phone tree;
  - Maintaining up-to-date websites;
  - Creating an e-mail listserv;
  - Pre-recording messages on a designated call-in phone number; or
  - Posting notices in frequently accessed places. Posters can be found at: http://www.cdc.gov/germstopper/materials.htm.

- **Assist people with physical, sensory, intellectual, or communication disabilities** by using alternative communication strategies. For example, provide links to the CDC Resources for the Deaf and Hard of Hearing at: http://www.cdc.gov/h1n1flu/deaf.htm.

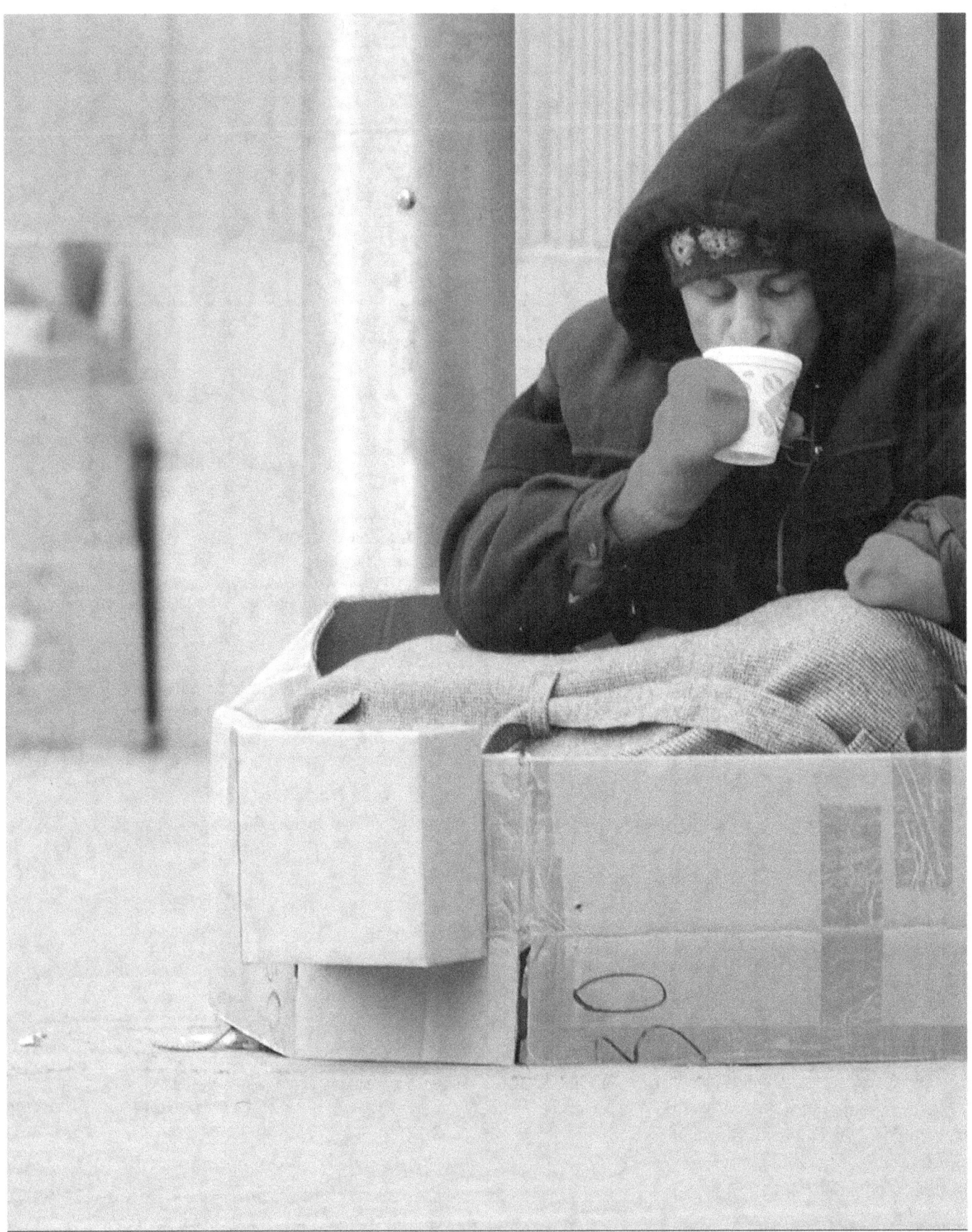

Vulnerable and Hard-to-Reach Populations

Some people have a higher risk of medical complications from seasonal and 2009 H1N1 flu, and CDC has prioritized these groups for vaccination. Many people, both targeted and not targeted for vaccination, face additional challenges during the 2009-2010 flu season because of their economic, social, or medical situations.

People in vulnerable and hard-to-reach populations may never receive important health messages because they are not connected to mainstream communication networks or because they cannot understand English. Others may be unable to afford healthcare or to access the services they need to stay healthy. Although vulnerable and hard-to-reach populations may vary from community to community, they may include:

- Low-income individuals and families;

- Non-English speakers;

- Homeless individuals and families;

- Shut-in or home-bound individuals.

- Migrant workers, immigrants, and refugees; and

- People with physical, sensory, mental health, intellectual, and cognitive disabilities;

What special challenges do vulnerable and hard-to-reach populations face?

- **Barriers to communication.** Inability to understand English, hear oral announcements, see directional signs, read written information, or access traditional forms of communication.

- **Specialized medical care.** Unstable, terminal, or contagious conditions requiring specialized care.

- **Requirements for independence in daily activities.** Need for consumable medical supplies (formula, bandages, etc.), medical equipment (wheelchairs, oxygen, etc.), and/or caregivers.

- **Supervision needs.** Eldercare or care for adults suffering from dementia, Alzheimer's disease, severe anxiety, etc.

- **Transportation barriers.** Inability to drive, limited or no access to a private vehicle, or requirements for accessible vehicles.

- **Economic or social dislocation.** Lack of economic resources and/or limited access to social support and mainstream communication networks.

What can my organization do to help vulnerable and hard-to-reach people in my community?

Your organization can provide programs and services critical to helping vulnerable and hard-to-reach individuals and families. Here are some suggestions:

- Identify which members of your community might need extra assistance.

- Translate documents and health materials into languages spoken by members of your community.

- Ensure that messages are simple and clear for low-literacy audiences.

- Develop a "necessities bank" to provide needed items to individuals who cannot afford them.

- Provide transportation for community members who can't drive or who rely on public transportation systems.

- Organize services for members needing assistance picking up medication, equipment, or supplies.

- Read Appendix C for an overview of an effective partnership to provide vaccine to vulnerable and hard-to-reach populations.

My organization supports homeless and emergency shelters. How can we protect the health of our clients, staff, and volunteers?

CDC has released specific guidance for homeless and emergency shelters, available at: http://www.cdc.gov/h1n1flu/guidance/homeless.htm. Some recommendations include:

- Minimizing contact between sick people and well people;

- Providing hand sanitizers and access to hand-washing facilities; and

- Staying informed about current guidance from CDC and your state or local health department.

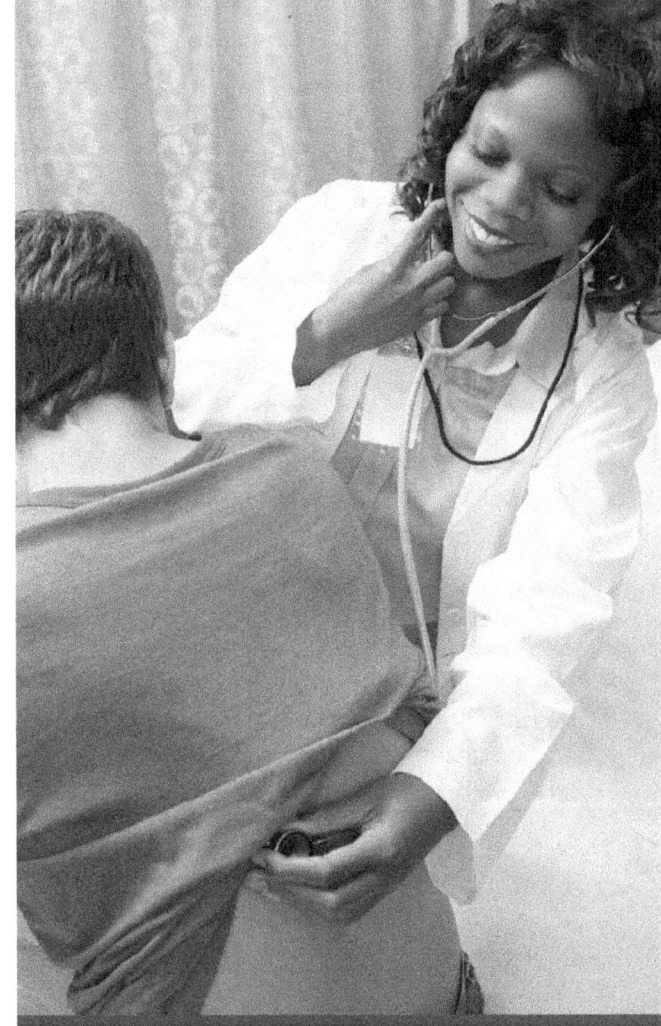

BOX 4: Parish nurses can play an important role in the flu response by:

- Organizing flu vaccination campaigns in their congregations;

- Helping people understand the vaccination target groups and encouraging those groups to get vaccinated;

- Providing information to community members on hygiene and healthy practices;

- Supporting individuals as they safely care for sick family members; and

- Caring for patients who require home care, especially those recently discharged by the hospital.

Participation in Community Response

How can my organization support increased needs for medical personnel?

During the 2009-2010 flu season, hospital staff may be overextended. Here are some steps that your organization can take to help meet the demand for medical personnel:

- **Check with your local hospital system and health department to see whether there are non-medical needs that volunteers from your organization can fill.** Many community members—interpreters, chaplains, office workers, legal advisors, and others—can fill key support positions.

- **Connect with the Medical Reserve Corps in your community.** Community-based Medical Reserve Corps (MRC) units work locally to organize volunteers (including physicians, nurses, pharmacists, and dentists) who donate their time and expertise to prepare for and respond to emergencies. MRC volunteers supplement existing emergency and public health resources. For more information, go to: http://www.medicalreservecorps.gov.

- **Engage parish nurses in flu response efforts** (see Box 4).

How can my organization's facility be used during the 2009 H1N1 flu response?

Talk with your local health department now to determine ways in which your volunteers and facilities might be useful during the response to 2009 H1N1 flu. For more information on using your building for vaccine distribution, see Section B.

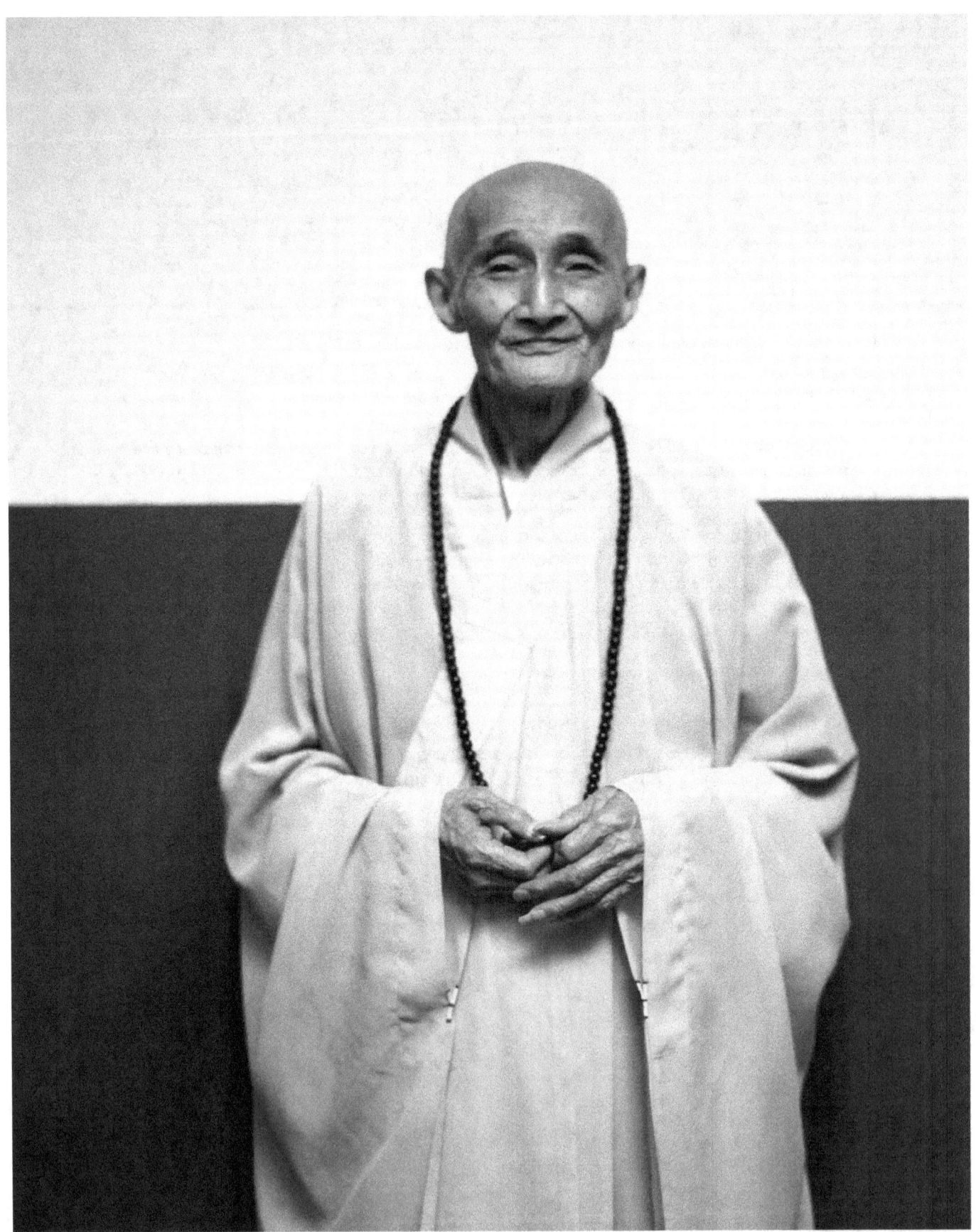

Meetings and Gatherings

Many faith-based and community groups hold services or meetings that bring people together. If the flu is causing more severe disease, CDC and your local health department may suggest that people avoid close contact with others and avoid attending large gatherings, a practice often called social distancing. These measures are intended to slow the spread of flu. Religious traditions and obligations may make it difficult to implement social distancing measures. However, faith-based and other community groups can do some specific things to help keep their members healthy.

What steps can leaders of religious services or community meetings take if there is an outbreak of flu in my community?

- To the extent possible, **make decisions in accordance with your state and local health departments about community gatherings and religious services** during widespread flu illness in your community. People should not be discouraged from gathering unless advised by public health officials.

- **Encourage people to wash hands often with soap and water.** If soap and water are not available, use an alcohol-based hand rub. If soap and water are not available and alcohol-based products are not allowed, other hand sanitizers that do not contain alcohol may be useful.

- **Remind people to cover their mouth and nose with a tissue when coughing or sneezing.** It may prevent those around them from getting sick.

- **Reduce crowding** as much as possible.

- **Identify which activities may increase the chance of spreading flu.** Work with your local health department to make decisions about changing or limiting these activities in order to help keep people healthy.
  - People gathering in close proximity may increase the risk of flu transmission.
  - Many religious services and community meetings involve a time of greeting or recognition by shaking hands or hugging. Encouraging interaction without physical contact and implementing social distancing measures may reduce the spread of flu in your community.
  - Some religious traditions and rituals emphasize eating and drinking from communal dishes and vessels. Flu transmission may be possible in these circumstances. If flu is circulating widely in your community, faith and community leaders may consider adjusting such practices in order to reduce the spread of flu. Check with your local or state health department and http://www.flu.gov.

- **Encourage people with flu-like illness to stay home.** The spread of flu may be decreased if people with flu-like illness stay home for at least 24 hours after they are free of fever without the use of fever-reducing medications.

- If there is widespread flu illness in your community, **discuss the risks of attending gatherings for those at high risk of medical complications from flu.** By avoiding gatherings, these individuals may reduce their risk of becoming ill with flu.

- **Provide alternative options and venues for participation whenever possible** for individuals who are ill, home-bound, or have a high risk of flu complications and will not be able to attend gatherings. See Section C on communication for more information.

- **Check** http://www.cdc.gov/h1n1flu/guidance/public_gatherings.htm for additional guidance on holding public gatherings, including religious services.

Should people travel during the 2009-2010 flu season?

Individuals and groups preparing for travel (including religious pilgrimages, retreats, holiday celebrations, and missionary trips) should stay informed on the latest news and travel advisories from CDC and the U.S. Department of State. Find this information at: http://www.flu.gov/individualfamily/travelers/index.html. Share this information with community members accordingly. Travelers who wish to minimize the transmission of flu should:

- **Follow local health recommendations, including movement restrictions;**

- **Practice healthy habits to help stop the spread of flu; and**

- **Follow these recommendations if the traveler becomes ill:**
  - Stay home or in a hotel room for at least 24 hours after becoming free of fever without the use of fever-reducing medicines.
  - Seek medical care if the traveler has severe illness or is at high risk of medical complications. Contact the U.S. Embassy or Consulate for help obtaining medical care.
  - Closely monitor the traveler's health after the traveler returns to the United States.

Mental Health and Stigma

How can my organization provide emotional comfort and support to my community during the 2009-2010 flu season?

- **Provide community members with support and stress relief activities.**

- **Utilize existing mental health materials and resources,** especially those focused on coping with 2009 HINI flu. See Appendix B for some resources.

- Encourage clergy, lay counselors, staff, and volunteers to **maintain their own psychological, emotional, and spiritual well-being.** Also, encourage them to seek help when needed.

- **Connect community members to existing mental health and counseling services in the community.** Check http://mentalhealth.samhsa.gov/databases/ for information on mental health services in your community.

How can my organization prevent and stop the spread of stigma around 2009 HINI flu?

Your organization plays an important role in reducing stigma. Stigma during the spring 2009 HINI flu outbreaks placed blame on certain people who contracted the disease and misrepresented how the disease was spread. Your organization can help to avoid stigma and blame while meeting people's real desire to avoid infection by:

- Delivering public health messages that address people's concerns;

- Dispelling rumors, misinformation, fear, and anxiety present in your community; and

- Modeling respectful and compassionate behavior when interacting with members of communities that are being stigmatized.

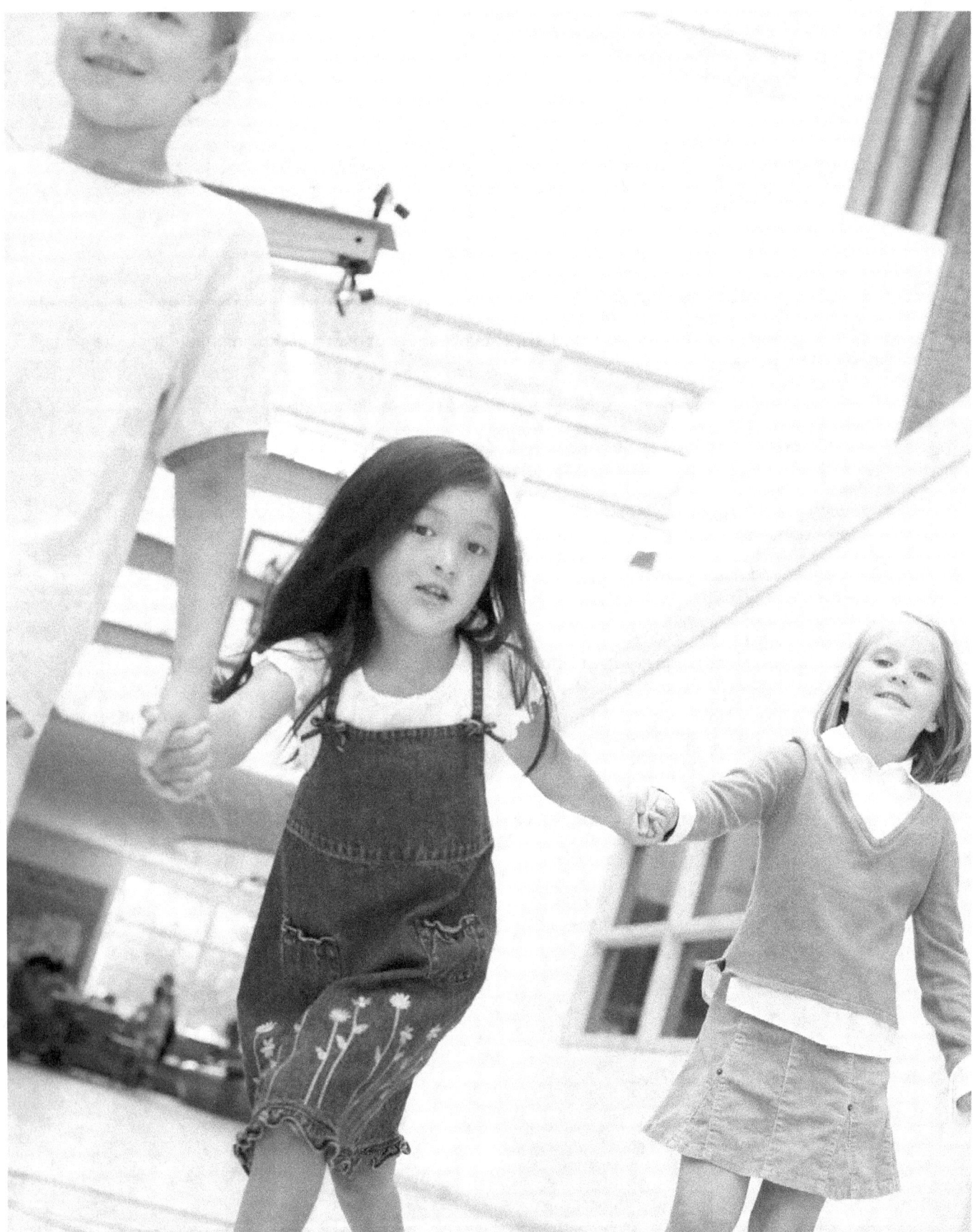

Childcare Organizations and Youth Programs

Will schools be dismissed during the 2009-2010 flu season?

The decision to dismiss students will be made locally. Find more information on schools and flu in the *Communication Toolkit for Schools*, available at: http://www.flu.gov/plan/school/toolkit.html.

How can my organization support efforts to prevent flu transmission in schools?

As part of your community's response, your organization can support schools as they endeavor to balance the risks of illness among students and staff with the benefits of keeping students in school. Your organization can encourage community members to plan to keep students home in the case of illness or a school dismissal. If it is not possible for parents to miss work or other commitments, your organization can organize emergency childcare options for these community members by matching these community members with a feasible childcare alternative.

Here are some steps your organization can take if school and public health officials make the local decision to dismiss schools:

- **Encourage children and teenagers to refrain from gathering in large groups** outside of school (for example, at shopping malls and other public places).

- **Make sure that children and youth can continue learning while out of school.** For example, your organization could:
  - Prepare learning materials, equipment, or books that could be useful for teaching and caring for children at home. Think about using local expertise and resources, like your organization's library or community members who are trained in education. See http://free.ed.gov for more information.
  - Make sure students have all that they need. Transport books, assignments, and completed work to and from the classroom and an ill child's home.

- **Provide nutritious meals to children normally receiving school lunches.** A good resource for creating healthy meals for infants, children, and adults is available at: http://www.fns.usda.gov/CND/Care/ProgramBasics/Meals/Meal_Patterns.htm.

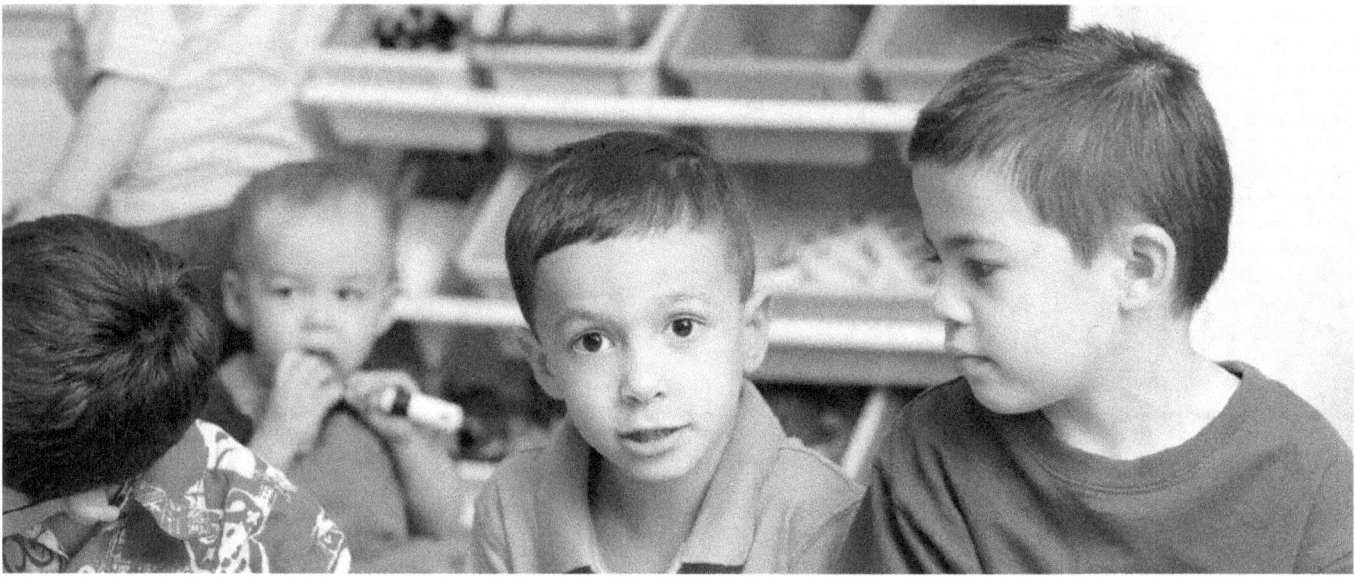

How can my childcare or after-school program support the 2009 H1N1 flu response?

Childcare and youth programs will be essential partners in protecting the public's health during the 2009-2010 flu season. CDC has developed specific guidance for Child Care and Early Childhood Programs during the 2009-2010 flu season. The guidance is available at: http://www.cdc.gov/h1n1flu/childcare/guidance.htm. Here are some steps you can take to help keep the children you serve healthy:

- **Stay home when sick.** Those with flu-like illness should stay home for at least 24 hours after they no longer have a fever or signs of a fever without the use of fever-reducing medicines. They should stay home even if they are using antiviral drugs. Early childhood programs, parents, or state and local health officials may elect to require longer periods of exclusion.

- **Separate ill students and staff.** Children and staff who appear to have flu-like illness should be sent to a room separate from others until they can be sent home. They should wear a surgical mask, if possible. Those caring for ill students should also wear protective gear.

- **Educate and encourage students to cover their mouth and nose with a tissue when they cough or sneeze.** Provide them with easy access to tissues. Remind them to cover coughs or sneezes using their elbow or shoulder instead of their hand when a tissue is not available.

- **Remind students to practice good hand hygiene.** Provide the time and supplies (easy access to running water and soap or hand sanitizers) for them to wash their hands as often as necessary.

- **Do routine cleaning.** Staff or volunteers should routinely clean areas that students and staff touch often. Special cleaning with bleach and other non-detergent-based cleaners is not necessary.

- **Increase distance between people.** Try developing innovative ways to separate students. These can be as simple as moving desks or workspaces farther apart or using larger rooms when available.

- **Get vaccinated against the flu.** All children and many staff in early childhood settings will fall within the target groups for the 2009 H1N1 flu vaccine.

- **Conduct daily health checks.** Early childhood providers observe all children for signs of illness and should talk with each child's parent or guardian.

- **Encourage early treatment for children and staff at high risk for flu complications.** Parents and staff should be encouraged to talk with their health care provider to determine whether they, or a member of their family, are at high risk for flu complications.

- **Consider selective early childhood program closures.** Work closely with your local health department to determine whether your early childhood program should be temporarily closed.

Work Environments

How should my organization's work environment change during the 2009-2010 flu season?

Your organization should be prepared for staff and volunteer absence during the upcoming flu season. Many members of your organization may need to stay home because they or their family members are sick or because schools and childcare centers are closed.

Here are some steps you can take to ensure that your organization continues to operate effectively:

- **Encourage sick staff and volunteers to stay home** and away from the workplace, and provide flexible leave or telework policies.

- **Encourage all employees and staff who are in target groups for 2009 H1N1 flu to get vaccinated.**

- **Encourage staff and volunteers to get the seasonal flu vaccine** in accordance with CDC recommendations.

- **Encourage early treatment for staff at high risk for flu complications.** Staff and volunteers at high risk for flu complications and parents of children younger than age 5 who become ill with flu-like illness should call their healthcare provider as soon as possible to determine whether they need antiviral treatment.

- **Display posters that remind employees about proper hand washing and covering coughs and sneezes.** These posters can be found on the following CDC website: http://www.cdc.gov/germstopper/materials.htm.

- **Provide facilities for hand washing** and/or hand sanitizers in common areas, like lobbies, corridors, and restrooms.

- **Routinely clean surfaces and items that are touched frequently.** Additional disinfection beyond routine cleaning is not necessary.

- **Prepare for staff and volunteers to stay home and plan ways for essential business functions to continue.** Cross-train staff to perform essential functions so that your organization can continue operating.

- **Plan for financial impacts** associated with 2009 H1N1 flu.

  - Budget: Consider the impact of 2009 H1N1 flu response and other unforeseen emergencies that can lead to a shortage of funds.

  - Charitable development strategies: Since many non-profit organizations rely on community giving to support their activities, they may want to use alternative means of receiving contributions, for example, by mail or internet.

- **Check CDC's** *Toolkit for Businesses and Employers* for more information on things you can do in the workplace to help keep your organization functioning and your employees healthy: http://www.flu.gov/plan/workplaceplanning/toolkit.html.

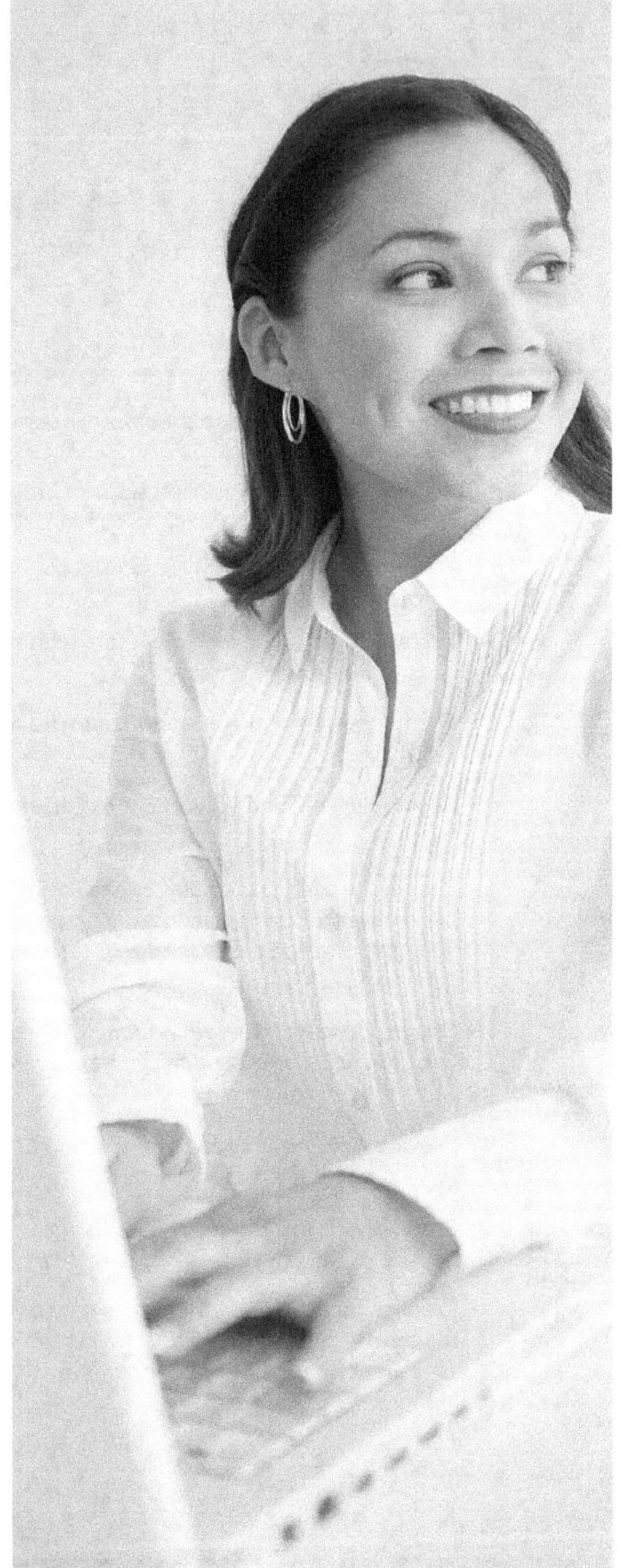

APPENDICES:

Appendix A: About Flu

Appendix B: Resources

Appendix C: Lessons Learned from the Minnesota
Immunization Networking Initiative (MINI):
Delivering Flu Vaccine in Non-traditional Settings

About Flu

How do I know the difference between 2009 H1N1 flu or seasonal flu?

It will be very hard to tell whether someone who is sick has 2009 H1N1 flu or seasonal flu. Public health officials and medical authorities do not recommend laboratory testing except in specific circumstances. Anyone who has flu-like symptoms should stay home and not go to work or school.

Symptoms of flu include fever or chills and cough or sore throat. Other possible symptoms include runny nose, body aches, headache, tiredness, diarrhea, or vomiting.

How do I recognize a fever or signs of a fever?

A fever is a temperature taken with a thermometer that is equal to or greater than 100 degrees Fahrenheit (38 degrees Celsius). If a sick person's temperature cannot be taken, look to see whether the person feels very warm, has a flushed appearance, is sweating, or is shivering.

Will there be a 2009 H1N1 flu vaccine?

Yes. The 2009 H1N1 flu vaccine is expected to be available for the public in October 2009. The seasonal flu vaccine will be available from early September 2009 onward.

Who is at high risk for medical complications from flu?

Anyone can get flu and can have serious problems from flu, though some groups are at higher risk for complications from seasonal or 2009 H1N1 flu. These include children younger than 5 years of age, pregnant women, people of any age with chronic health conditions, and people 65 years of age and older.

Medical conditions associated with a higher risk of flu-related complications include: chronic pulmonary (including asthma), cardiovascular (except hypertension), renal, hepatic, cognitive, neurologic/neuromuscular, hematologic, or metabolic disorders (including diabetes mellitus) and immunosuppression (including HIV and immunosuppression caused by medications).

Individuals should talk with their healthcare provider to determine whether they are at higher risk for flu complications, especially if they have been in close contact with others who are sick with flu or flu-like illness.

If people in these groups get flu-like symptoms, they should seek treatment—including antiviral treatment—from a healthcare provider within 48 hours.

What can I do to protect myself and others from getting sick?

There are some key things that you can do right now to help keep you and your family healthy.

Everyday steps to protect your health:

- Cover your nose and mouth with a tissue when you cough or sneeze. Throw the tissue in the trash after you use it. If a tissue is unavailable, cough or sneeze into your shoulder or elbow instead of your hands.

- Wash your hands often with soap and warm water for at least 20 seconds, especially after you cough or sneeze. You can also use alcohol-based hand sanitizers.

- Avoid touching your eyes, nose, or mouth. Germs spread this way.

- Try to avoid close contact with sick people.

- Keep sick children at home.

- If you have flu-like symptoms (fever with cough or sore throat), stay home for at least 24 hours after you are free of fever without the use of fever-reducing medications like Tylenol®. This step is to help stop spreading the virus to others.

Some other important actions during the 2009-2010 flu season:

- Get the seasonal flu vaccine if recommended by CDC or if you want to reduce your chance of getting the flu.

- Get vaccinated for 2009 H1N1 flu if you are in one of the target groups. Others may be able to get the vaccine after local demand among target groups has been met.

- Follow public health advice and guidance. For example, avoid close contact with others attending large gatherings of people (often called social distancing measures).

- Be prepared in case you get sick and need to stay home for a week or so. Keep a supply of over-the-counter medicines, alcohol-based hand sanitizers, tissues, and other related items so that you do not need to make trips outside your home while you are sick and contagious.

- Stay informed by checking with your local health department or http://www.flu.gov for updates related to staying healthy.

Resources

1. The most up-to-date, comprehensive information on 2009 HINI flu:
   www.flu.gov
   or
   www.cdc.gov/HINIflu

2. The Centers for Disease Control and Prevention (CDC) Hotline:
   1-800-CDC-INFO (1-800-232-4636)
   Available in English and Spanish, 24 hours a day, 7 days a week.
   TTY: 1-888-232-6348.
   Email questions to: cdcinfo@cdc.gov.

3. HHS Center for Faith-based and Neighborhood Partnerships:
   http://www.hhs.gov/partnership
   200 Independence Avenue, S.W.
   Washington, DC 20201
   Phone: (202) 358-3595   Fax: (202) 401-3463

4. World Health Organization (WHO) Influenza Website:
   http://www.who.int/csr/disease/swineflu/en/index.html

5. To contact your state or local health department, call 311 or visit: http://www.apha.org/about/Public+Health+Links/LinksStateandLocalHealthDepartments.htm

6. The Faith-Based & Community Organizations Pandemic Influenza Preparedness Checklist (a checklist for pandemic planning): http://www.pandemicflu.gov/plan/community/faithcomchecklist.html)

7. National Voluntary Organizations Active in Disaster:
   http://www.nvoad.org

8. The American Red Cross (a resource on coping and emotional health during HINI): http://www.redcross.org/www-files/Documents/pdf/Preparedness/SwineHINIFluCopingFactSheet.pdf?utm_source=BRCR&utm_medium=PDF&utm_campaign=Flu_CopingTips

9. National Institute of Mental Health http://www.nimh.nih.gov/health/publications/index.shtml

Lessons Learned from the Minnesota Immunization Networking Initiative (MINI): Delivering Flu Vaccine in Non-traditional Settings

Why should local or state health departments build vaccination partnerships with community and faith-based organizations (CFBOs)?

- Faith communities and grassroots community organizations have established credibility in their respective communities, trusted leadership, and knowledge of and relationships with hard-to-reach populations, such as vulnerable adults, immigrants, and special needs persons.

- Many CFBOs have an existing infrastructure of health promotion through the work of a faith community registered nurse or a health cabinet/committee.

Why should CFBOs collaborate with public health or state departments of health?

- By providing a facility site for vaccinations, faith communities and other community organizations can fulfill a mission to serve people in need.

- Faith communities can model commitment to wellness for the whole person by hosting flu vaccinations. They can demonstrate that caring for the physical body is an honorable part of their faith tradition.

Getting Started: Influenza vaccinations in non-traditional settings

Community needs/strengths assessment: Contact the local public health department, the immunizations department at your local or state health department, and the local Immunization Action Coalition. Look at health disparities data in your region, including numbers of uninsured, underserved, and those without a medical home. Gather facts, information, and advice. Find out who is currently providing vaccinations in your locale (health departments, visiting nurses, and healthcare companies that contract with businesses for employee vaccination).

Build the collaboration: Identify and invite potential partners to an organizational meeting, including representatives from state and local public health agencies, faith communities, service providers, non-profit collaborations, local coalitions, and networks. Present information that documents the need for vaccine provision through non-traditional sites. Locate an organization or agency that could provide healthcare professionals and vaccine. Discuss roles and responsibilities for the different members of the collaboration, including a clear leadership structure.

Vaccine delivery requirements: A licensed healthcare provider with a doctor's orders (standing orders); liability insurance; licensed healthcare professionals (nurses and medical assistants); vaccine (multi-dose vials, individual syringes, or intranasal) and supplies (syringes, gauze, and bandages); and printed materials such as consent forms, Vaccination Information Statements (VIS), and privacy statements. Find CDC's protocol for delivery of vaccinations in non-traditional settings at: http://www.cdc.gov/mmwr/preview/mmwrhtml/rr4901a1.htm and information on the Public Readiness and Emergency Preparedness Act at: http://www.hhs.gov/disasters/emergency/manmadedisasters/bioterorism/medication-vaccine-qa.html

Roles/responsibilities: The **program manager** will coordinate meetings (planning, coordination, and evaluation); act as liaison to public health/state department of health and the healthcare provider(s); solicit financial support through grant applications; and if necessary, solicit donations of vaccine (excess vaccine is typically available in December from pharmaceutical companies, clinics, drug stores, etc.). Appoint a **site coordinator** for each participating community partner organization who will coordinate with the program manager to schedule sites and arrange for facility use. Each host site will be responsible for necessary interpreters, volunteers, and publicity.

Appendix C was authored by Patricia Peterson, Faith Community Outreach Manager, Fairview Health Services, Minneapolis, MN. If you would like to obtain more information, please contact her by phone at (612) 672-2807 or email (ppeters1@fairview.org).